Drop Acid
The New Amazing Study of Uric Acid

By

Norman S. Watson

Table of contents

Introduction

With regards to losing weight, you need to identify your remarkable way and how your body utilizes the fuel you give it. While that might sound excessively confounded, it's not when you figure continuous glucose monitors (CGMs). These devices assist you with looking past the number on the scale to comprehend your general well-being and how your body's chemicals manage glucose.

The imperfections of the calorie deficit model of weight reduction can be envisioned by imagining the human body as a vehicle: The motor is our cells, the gas tank is our fat stores, and the fuel inside the tank is given by the food we eat. As we drive the vehicle along, the motor (cells) consumes fuel (fat) to keep the vehicle moving. By eating food, we "top up" the tank as we go, keeping it from drying up. In this similarity, to drain our gas tank (fat stores), we can place less fuel in the tank (eat fewer calories) or drive the vehicle quicker (exercise more). It's difficult to eliminate stress, yet we can hose its effects by executing a routine that integrates regular exercise and unwinding procedures. We can't do everything at once, it doesn't come about by accident more or less, and unquestionably not with craze diets and exercise programs. Yet, on the off chance that we address nourishment, work out, rest, stress, and hydration slowly and carefully, the chances of achievement increment hugely." remain tuned for these uncommon tips for extraordinary well-being.

Chapter 1
Basic of Uric Acid:

Uric acid is a toxic water in the body. At times, uric acid can develop in the joints and tissues, causing a scope of medical issues. These include gout, a type of arthritis.

Uric acid is a compound made when the body separates substances called purines. Purines are ordinarily delivered in the body and are additionally tracked down in certain food varieties and beverages. Food sources with high content of purines include liver, anchovies, mackerel, dried beans and peas, and beer.

Most uric acid breaks up in the blood and goes to the kidneys. From that point, it drops in urine. Assuming your body delivers an excessive amount of uric acid or doesn't eliminate enough of it, you can become ill. A raised degree of uric acid in the blood is known as hyperuricemia.
Uric acid is orchestrated predominantly in the liver, digestion tracts, and the vascular endothelium as the final result of

an exogenous pool of purines, and endogenously from damaged, dying, and dead cells, by which nucleic acids, adenine, and guanine, are reduced into uric acid. Referencing uric acid produces fear since it is the laid out etiological specialist of the serious, intense, and constant fiery arthritis, and gout and is embroiled in the commencement and progress of the metabolic disorder. However, uric acid is the dominating enemy of oxidant particles in plasma and is essential and adequate for the acceptance of type 2 resistant reactions. These properties might make sense of its defensive likely in neurological and irresistible illnesses, mostly schistosomiasis. The essential defensive capability of uric acid against blood-borne microorganisms and neurological and immune system sicknesses is yet to be laid out.

High uric acid levels in the body can make crystals of uric acid structure, prompting gout. A few food and beverages that are high in purines can build the degree of uric acid. It is surprising to have low uric acid levels, however, it is conceivable if an individual passes an excess of uric acid out of their body as waste.

Having some uric acid in the blood is ordinary. Notwithstanding, if uric acid levels go above or under a healthy range, this can bring about medical conditions. High uric acid levels can expand the gamble of gout.

What is gout?

Gout is a typical type of provocative joint inflammation that is exceptionally difficult. Most times, it affects one joint at a time (frequently the huge toe joint). There are times when symptoms deteriorate, known as flares, and times when there are no symptoms, known as remission. Repeated bouts of gout can prompt gouty joint inflammation, a deteriorating type of joint inflammation.

There is no solution for gout, yet you can successfully treat and deal with the condition with medicine and self-administration methodologies.
Gout flares start suddenly and can last days or weeks. These flares are trailed by extensive stretches of remission — weeks, months, or

years — without symptoms before another flare starts. Gout for the most part happens in just a single joint at a time. It is much of the time tracked down in the huge toe. Alongside the large toe, joints that are generally impacted are the lesser toe joints, the lower leg, and the knee.

Symptoms in the affected joint(s) may include:
Paint, normally extraordinary
Swelling
Redness
Heat

What causes gout?

Gout is brought about by a condition known as hyperuricemia, where there is an excess of uric acid in the body. The body makes uric acid when it separates purines, which are found in your body, and the food varieties you eat. At the point when there is a lot of uric acid in the body, uric acid crystals (monosodium urate) can develop in joints, fluids, and tissues inside the body. Hyperuricemia doesn't necessarily cause gout, and hyperuricemia without gout symptoms won't be necessary for treatment.

How is gout treated?

Gout can be successfully treated and dealt with with clinical treatment and self-administration techniques. Your primary care provider might advice a clinical therapy scheme to deal with the pain of a flare. Treatment for flares comprises nonsteroidal anti-inflammatory drugs

(NSAIDs) like ibuprofen, steroids, and the mitigating drug colchicine.

Forestall future flares. Making changes to your eating routine and way of life, for example, shedding pounds, restricting liquor, and eating less purine-rich food (like red meat or organ meat), may assist with forestalling future attacks. Changing or halting meds related to hyperuricemia (like diuretics) may likewise help.

Forestall tophi and kidney stones from framing because of constantly elevated degrees of uric acid. Tophi are hard, and uric acid is stored under the skin. For individuals with regular intense flares or persistent gout, specialists might prescribe preventive treatment to bring down uric acid levels in the blood utilizing drugs like allopurinol, febuxostat, and pegloticase. Notwithstanding clinical treatment, you can deal with your gout with self-administration methodologies. Self-administration is what you do every day to deal with your condition and remain solid, such as settling on a sound way of life decisions.

The simple meaning of uric acid:

Uric acid is a definitive catabolite of purine digestion in people and higher primates. It is a feeble natural acid that under physiologic circumstances exists chiefly as a monosodium salt. At a pH under 5.75, as may happen in the urine, the dominating structure is nonionized uric acid. The solvency of monosodium urate is multiple times more prominent than uric acid in fluid arrangements. This solvency differential gives the remedial reasoning to alkalinization of the urine pH to more prominent than 6.0 in patients shaping uric acid stones.

The furthest reaches of plasma uric acid might be characterized by a factual reach in a typical populace. Epidemiologic examinations in the US have commonly acknowledged 7.0 mg/dl as far as possible in grown-up men and 6.0 mg/dl in ladies.

The physiochemical meaning of hyperuricemia might be viewed as

7.0 mg/dl estimated by the particular uricase strategy. This addresses the dissolvability furthest reaches of urate in plasma at 37°C. Levels past 7.0 outcome in supersaturated arrangements that are inclined to gem development.

Uric acid levels are affected by age and sex. Preceding pubescence, the typical serum uric acid is 3.6 mg/dl for guys and females. Following adolescence, values ascend to grown-up levels with ladies commonly 1 mg/dl not as much as men. This lower level in ladies reflects an estrogen-related improvement of renal urate leeway and vanishes at menopause. Numerous extra factors, including exercise, diet, medications, and condition of hydration, may bring about transient vacillations of uric acid levels.

Serum uric acid mirrors the connections of four significant cycles: dietary purine consumption, endogenous purine digestion, urinary urate discharge, and gastrointestinal uricolysis.

The regular American eating regimen might give a critical

purine load. People don't rely upon exogenous purines to act as antecedents of tissue nucleic acids, and practically this dietary part is directly changed over into uric acid. Xanthine oxidase, the chemical answerable for the change of oxypurines to uric acid, is tracked down in overflow in the liver and the mucosa of the small digestive tract. Most dietary nucleic acids are ingested as nucleoproteins and can be metabolized to uric acid at the level of the stomach mucosa.

Historically, the cornerstone of antihyperuricemic therapy has been dietary management. However, even strict purine-free diets only modestly lower serum uric acid levels, often by around 1 mg/dl. The therapeutic significance of nutrition has received less attention as a result of the development of effective antihyperuricemic medications. However, some foods, like organ meats, are high in purines and, if consumed in large enough doses, can significantly alter serum uric acid levels.

De novo biosynthesis and the degradation of tissue nucleic acids are the sources of endogenous purines. Isotopic dilution techniques must be used on patients who are extremely purine-deficient in their diets to determine the true rate of endogenous purine turnover. Measuring a 24-hour urine collection for uric acid is a more realistic technique in patients with a normal renal function who are not receiving uricosuric medications. This gives a rough idea of how quickly purine is produced. A generally acknowledged upper limit for uric acid excretion on purine-restricted diets is 600 mg/24 hours. The restriction is increased to 800 mg/24 hours on an unrestricted diet.

Occasionally, people with primary hyperuricemia excrete too much uric acid. Only a small percentage of these patients had a particular regulatory enzyme deficiency found. Accelerated urine excretion of uric acid is linked to hyperuricemia related to hematologic conditions with increased cellular turnover, such as hemolytic and myeloproliferative illnesses, which are linked to an increase in uric acid excretion from the urine. In these illnesses, the rate of purine production is increased to make up for the faster turnover of nucleic acids. Finally, several exogenous compounds, like fructose and methylene blue, may promote purine production. Two-thirds to three-quarters of daily losses are accounted for by the kidney, which is the primary site for uric acid elimination. The four processes of glomerular filtration, proximal tubular reabsorption, secretion, and postsecretory reabsorption are thought to work together to regulate and create excretion. Most people with primary hyperuricemia and gout show a deficiency in the kidneys' ability to handle uric acid. The development of hyperuricemia in these patients might, in theory, be attributed to any component of the model failing. At this time, The defect's precise location is still a problem.

Secondary hyperuricemia can result from renal failure and a decreased glomerular filtration rate. Through several processes, including an increase in tubular reabsorption, diuretics raise serum uric acid levels. Several organic acids, including lactate, betahydroxybutyrate, and acetoacetate, may impede the secretory pathway for uric acid. This explains some of the hyperuricemia present in lactic acidosis and diabetic ketoacidosis. Less than 2.5 gm/day of salicylates disrupt the secretory system and increase serum uric acid levels. Higher doses cause urate diuresis and lower serum uric acid levels by inhibiting urate absorption.

The digestive process known as intestinal uricolysis, which is carried out by enzymes of the gut bacterial flora, generally eliminates between 25 and 30 percent of uric acid. Through gastrointestinal secretions, such as saliva, bile, gastric, pancreatic, and intestinal fluids, uric acid enters the intestines. It is unknown whether intestinal uricolysis failure can result in hyperuricemia. In patients with renal failure, the role of intestine degradation increases and may be responsible for up to 80% of urate elimination.

The unspoken link between diabetes and dementia that characterizes our contemporary diseases:

Both the prevalences of diabetes and dementia are rising globally, especially among older individuals. Between 13 and 20% of persons with dementia have diabetes. Dementia may harm diabetes control and diabetic self-care. Knowing the most effective diabetes treatment strategies for PLWD in various contexts and at different stages of the disease. The ultimate goal is to identify potential interventions that need further assessment and to construct an explanatory account or program theory about "what works" in the management of diabetes in persons in what environment.

Diabetes: Diabetes is a condition in which your body's cells are unable to absorb sugar (glucose) and use it as fuel. As a result, your bloodstream begins to accumulate additional sugar.

Diabetes that is not properly managed can have catastrophic

effects and harm several body organs and tissues, including the heart, kidneys, eyes, and nerves. When a person develops diabetes, their body struggles to keep blood glucose levels at normal levels. Our bodies primary source of energy is glucose, a type of sugar. Blood glucose levels that are unhealthy might cause both immediate and long-term health problems.

Dementia: is the loss of cognitive abilities, such as thinking, remembering, and reasoning, to the point where it significantly affects a person's ability to carry out daily tasks. Some dementia patients have emotional instability and personality changes. The potency of dementia differs from the mildest phase, when it is just beginning to interfere with a someone's ability to act, to the most severe level, when the individual must completely rely on others for basic daily activities up. You might experience a range of emotions if you recently learned that you or a loved one has dementia. You can feel astonished, terrified of the future, or unhappy about potential life

changes or opportunities you
might lose out on. Even when
your symptoms have a reason,
you might feel relieved.
Dementia is primarily treated with
supportive care. Prescription
drugs cannot stop or reverse the
process. A disciplined routine,
consistent exercise, and
maintaining social engagements
can all be helpful.

- Note: dementia and diabetes
  are related. Alzheimer's
  disease and vascular
  dementia are just two
  examples of the cognitive

impairment that type 2 diabetics are more likely to face.

Cognitive impairment encompasses a range of problems, including difficulties with focus, learning new things, remembering details, and making judgments.

Because diabetes and dementia are complicated diseases, a person's life expectancy may be impacted by a variety of circumstances. For instance, a person with diabetes who does not adequately control their glucose levels or take care of themselves is likely to live shorter than a person whose diabetes is well-managed.

Many people who have diabetes and dementia also have other chronic illnesses, which can make their health situation much more difficult.

Diabetes and dementia patients need specialized care and management. Therefore, it's crucial to create a thorough treatment plan in collaboration with a doctor.

To lower their risk of type 2 diabetes, people can make

lifestyle changes. The actions to take could be any of the following, depending on their existing way of life:

- Weight loss:
For those who are overweight, dccrcasing 5-7% of their weight may lower their chance of developing diabetes.
- Moving more:
Aim for at least 30 minutes of physical activity each day, five days a week.
- Consuming a balanced diet:
Whole grains, fruits, vegetables, and lean protein should all be

staples in a well-balanced diet. Limiting the consumption of processed meals and sugary beverages is recommended.

There are currently no effective treatments or preventions for dementia like Alzheimer's. But if necessary, following the advice above might be beneficial.

There is a chance that diabetes and dementia will co-occur. Dementia seems to be more likely in people with diabetes. This might be because insulin helps to create the amyloid plaques that are a defining feature of Alzheimer's disease in the brain.

Diabetes with dementia management might be challenging. No one solution works for everyone, but working with a doctor to create an all-encompassing treatment plan is crucial. It's also essential to create a supportive environment for the patient and their caregivers.

A healthy lifestyle can lower one's risk of developing diabetes. However, dementia cannot be prevented using known methods.

Chapter 2
How sleep, salt, and seafood relate to uric Acid

Sleep: Loss of sleep or irregular sleep-wake patterns have been linked to metabolic impairments. Sleep is a critical factor in determining metabolic homeostasis. It has been demonstrated that sleep deprivation and sleep-wake cycle disruptions activate proteolytic pathways, which may change the equilibrium between protein synthesis and degradation and favor catabolism. Proteins are consequently degraded into their by-products, such as purines, which are then converted into uric acid. Only one study has looked at correlations between subjective sleep duration and SUA levels so far, and it produced no conclusive findings.

Shorter sleep duration was linked to greater uric acid levels, whereas poor sleep quality was linked to lower levels.

Salt: According to reports, cardiovascular illness is linked to high salt intake and high uric acid (UA) levels. In this study, the effects of daily salt intake and UA on the risk of developing prehypertension were examined. A high-salt diet has been proven to reduce uric acid levels in the blood, a known gout trigger. When prehypertensive subjects consume salt, urinary UA excretion increases. Prehypertension risk is increased when serum UA levels are high and salt intake is high.

Seafood: Although it's advised to eat a lot of fish as part of a balanced diet, persons who have gout should be aware that some seafood might raise uric acid levels in the blood and perhaps aggravate their condition. Anchovies, codfish, haddock, herring, mackerel, mussels, sardines, scallops, and trout all have high purine contents. Purines can likewise be found regularly in fish and other seafood. Scallops, oily fishes, herring, and mackerel are the bad offenders if you have gout. Seafood and shellfish should be avoided due to their high purine content to reduce the risk of a gout flare.When consumed in moderation, certain fish, such as salmon, sole, tuna, catfish, red snapper, tilapia, flounder, and whitefish, are lower in purine than other varieties. If you do not consume other purine-rich foods, (two to three times per week)Seafood, such as oysters, lobster, crab, and shrimp, should only be consumed infrequently due to their high purine content.

Chapter 3
Dietary changes to reduce uric acid levels:

The practice gained more support after the discovery of purines in 1884, and consumers began to receive regular warnings against eating otherwise healthy foods like fish, vegetables, and fruit because they also contained the chemical.

However, knowledge of the production of uric acid has significantly increased in recent years, and many of the plant-based high-purine meals that were formerly prohibited from ingestion are now regarded as safe.

Uric acid is excreted from the body after purine-rich foods have been digested. Purines are chemical substances that are broken down in the body and are composed of carbon and nitrogen atoms. When we consume too many purine-rich meals, our bodies are unable to digest them, which raises the amounts of uric acid in our bodies. Patients with high uric acid levels must be extremely careful with their diet and eating habits. You should also prevent eating too much fat, as this may impair your body's ability to expel uric acid, in addition to avoiding foods high in purines.

A higher than normal uric acid level in the blood can cause gout. It's crucial to keep an eye on your eating habits if you want to avoid this ailment. With a balanced diet and the appropriate medication, you might be able to keep your uric acid levels within the normal range. The foods listed below should be a part of your diet if you want to keep your uric acid levels within normal ranges.

What to consume…

• Water:
Yet more justification for
drinking enough of it every day.
Water aids in the body's removal
of impurities, particularly
excessive uric acid. So, drink at
least 8 to 9 glasses of water daily.

• freshly made veggie juices:
 Make sure to combine the carrot
liquid with the beet and cucumber
juices. High blood uric acid levels
can be treated successfully with
this remedy.

- Low-fat dairy products: Including low-fat dairy products in your diet is another strategy to treat elevated uric acid. To reduce the levels of uric acid in your blood, choose low-fat milk and curd.

- Lime:
Including lime juice in your diet regularly will help lower your uric acid levels since it contains citric acid, a uric acid solvent. Day to day, drink a glass of water with a bisection of lime juice squeezed into it.
nutrient-dense foods: Including foods that are high in dietary fiber

also lowers blood levels of uric acid. They assist your kidneys to remove extra uric acid from your body by absorbing it from the bloodstream. Increase your intake of dietary soluble fibers such as oats, apples, oranges, broccoli, pears, strawberries, blueberries, cucumbers, celery, carrots, and barley if you have been diagnosed with elevated uric acid.

- Bananas:

Eat bananas since having them in your diet helps to reduce high uric acid levels.

- broccoli, cucumbers, and tomatoes:

Before taking your meal, eat broccoli, tomatoes, and cucumbers. This is the greatest way to prevent your blood from becoming too acidic from uric acid buildup. Their alkaline state helps to maintain blood uric acid levels.

plus a lot more….

Practices to Avoid

• Surgery foods and beverages Recent research has revealed that sugar can also have a role in the development of elevated uric acid, which is typically associated with a diet heavy in protein. Table sugar, corn syrup, and high fructose corn syrup are the most prevalent added sugars. Particularly fructose causes a rise in uric acid levels. It is best to examine the labels of food items for sugar before buying.Eat more natural foods and fewer refined packaged meals if you want to cut back on your sugar intake.

- Avoid alcohol:

Have you ever noticed that drinking alcohol increases the frequency with which you use the restroom? Alcohol causes dehydration and raises uric acid levels. This occurs because alcohol is being filtered out of the blood by your kidney instead of uric acid and other toxins.

Take control of your insulin levels:

High amounts of uric acid and weight gain might result from an excess of insulin in the body. It is a fine decision to get your insulin levels checked when you seek medical attention, even if you do not have diabetes mellitus.

How to Control Your Metabolism:

The process of turning the food and liquids we consume into

energy is called metabolism. Our bodies require energy to continue internal processes even when we are at rest (blood circulation, muscle repair, breathing, producing hormones, etc.)Your metabolism determines how many calories your body needs to perform these essential physiological processes.

The concept of "rapid" and "slow" metabolisms refers to the different ways in which each of our bodies handles this process. You will burn more calories both at rest and when you are active if your metabolism is "high" (or fast).

You'll need to consume more calories to maintain your weight if you have a high metabolism. One explanation for why some people can eat more than others without gaining weight is because a person with a "low" (or slow) metabolism will expend fewer calories when at rest and during activity, requiring them to consume fewer calories overall. There are several quick and simple methods to speed up metabolism, many of which only require minor dietary and lifestyle adjustments.

Here are some simple methods to speed up your metabolism:
1. Consume a lot of protein at each meal.
Your metabolism may briefly rise after eating for a few hours.

The thermic effect of food is what we refer to as this (TEF). The extra calories needed to digest, absorb, and utilize the nutrients in your food are what lead to it.

The greatest increase in TEF is due to protein. 20 to 30 percent of the useable energy in dietary protein must be used for metabolism, compared to 0 to 3% for lipids and 5 to 10% for carbohydrates.

You may increase your metabolism and burn more calories by eating more protein. Additionally, it may contribute to your feeling more satisfied and help you avoid overeating.

2. Consume more water

People who opt for water over sugary beverages frequently have better success with weight loss and weight maintenance.

This is because sugary drinks include calories, therefore

switching to water automatically lowers your calorie consumption. Water consumption, however, may potentially momentarily accelerate your metabolism. Water consumption might help you maintain your weight loss. It assists in filling you up before meals and momentarily speeds up your metabolism.

3. Perform an energetic workout. Quick and extremely intense bursts of activity are used in high-intensity interval training (HIIT). Even after your workout is over, if this form of exercise is safe for you, it can help you burn

additional fat by raising your metabolic rate.

Start with a modality you are currently comfortable with, like biking or jogging.Adding a few high-intensity sessions to your regular exercise program can speed up your metabolism and aid in fat loss.

4. Have a restful night's sleep
Obesity risk is significantly increased when people don't get enough sleep. This may be influenced by the negative effects of sleep loss on metabolism. A higher risk of developing type 2 diabetes has been associated with

both insulin resistance and elevated blood sugar levels, both of which have been connected to sleep deprivation.

This may help to explain why many sleep-deprived persons frequently feel hungry and may struggle to lose weight when doing so is their objective.

Lack of sleep can alter your metabolism, alter how you metabolize sugar, and interfere with the hormones that control your appetite.

Chapter 4:
The Fructose Myth

Fructose is one of the two main ingredients in added sugar, along with glucose.

Some medical professionals think fructose is worse than glucose, at least when ingested in excess.

50% of table sugar is made up of simple sugar fructose (sucrose). Glucose, which is the primary energy source for your body's cells, is also a component of table sugar.

But before fructose can be utilized by the body, the liver must transform it into glucose. Since the dawn of civilization, free fructose and sucrose have most likely been a staple of the human diet. They are naturally occurring substances found in fruits, vegetables, and honey. However, until the eighteenth century, when sugar became widely accessible at a low cost because of colonial trade, fructose consumption remained quite low. It's interesting to note how closely sweetened beverages—first tea, coffee, and chocolate in the nineteenth century, then sodas at the start of the twentieth—were associated with sugar consumption.

Numerous research studies and publications have been written and published since there has been a resurgence in interest in fructose-containing caloric sweeteners (FCCS), yet the debate persists. However, several health organizations came to the conclusion that added sugar consumption should be substantially limited to less than 5% of total energy.

Reasons Why Fructose Is Bad for You

The body processes glucose and fructose quite differently.

Every cell in the body can utilize glucose, but only the liver can digest fructose in large quantities. When a person eats a diet that is high in calories and high in fructose, their liver becomes strained and starts turning the extra fructose in their diet into fat. Most scientists believe that consuming excessive amounts of fructose may have a significant role in many of the most severe diseases that currently exist.

Among them are type II diabetes, heart disease, cancer, and obesity. Many health experts believe that high fructose intake is a major cause of metabolic issues.

The Negative Effects of Too Much Fructose

Although high fructose is certainly bad, its impacts on health remain debatable. However, there is a sizable body of evidence supporting the worries.

Consuming excessive amounts of added sugars that contain fructose may:

deteriorate the lipid makeup of
your blood.

Fructose may raise VLDL
cholesterol levels, which could
lead to heart disease by causing
fat to build up around in the
organs.

a rise in uric acid levels,
ultimately results in gout and high
blood pressure

cause the liver to accumulate fat,
which could result in non-
alcoholic fatty liver disease

The appetite-suppressing effects
of glucose outweigh those of

fructose. Therefore, it might encourage binge eating. Overindulging in fructose may result in leptin resistance, which would disrupt the body's ability to regulate body fat and lead to obesity.

Note that not all of this has been rigorously demonstrated in research. The data is still there, though, and in the upcoming years and decades, more studies will provide a clearer picture. Numerous studies indicate that a high fructose diet may increase the risk of developing chronic diseases in people.

how uric acid heightens the danger:

The global epidemic of metabolic syndrome is associated with both a considerable rise in total fructose intake and an increase in blood uric acid (in the form of table sugar and high-fructose corn syrup). Uric acid is increased by fructose, and this acid prevents nitric oxide from becoming bioavailable. We proposed that fructose-induced hyperuricemia may play a harmful role in metabolic syndrome because insulin needs nitric oxide to drive glucose absorption.

Most people are aware of how sugar contributes to weight gain. Obesity and related illnesses like diabetes and heart disease are influenced by eating too much sugar. Additionally, consuming too much high fructose corn syrup, which is present in processed foods and sodas, can cause severe gout. Gout is yet another health danger to be aware of, especially given that the typical American consumes 22 to 30 tablespoons of sugar every day.

Purines are a class of chemical substances that are released as fructose is broken down by the body. Uric acid, which causes gout and forms painful crystals in the joints, is created when purines are broken down. Your uric acid levels increase minutes after consuming high fructose corn syrup-sweetened soda.

Because dietary fructose is primarily metabolized by the liver and little fructose reaches systemic blood circulation, it may be regarded as a naturally occurring poison. Along with several other compounds created during fructose metabolism, uric acid has the potential to be hazardous. Regardless of the source of the fructose, such as whether it comes from an artificial sweetener, fruit juice, or whole fruit, the amount of uric acid released is based on the amount of fructose consumed. The kidneys expel two-thirds of the uric acid produced each day in the form of urine, with the remaining one-third passing via the small intestine (the third kidney) in the digestive fluids. Given that the symptoms of gout, which are caused by elevated serum uric acid, are obvious, it is expected that herbal remedies would have created effective treatments for the condition. However, it may come as a surprise to learn that the same herbs may also play a part in the management of metabolic syndrome.

The impact of dietary fructose intake on uric acid and the development of gout or metabolic syndrome is not currently addressed in recommendations. Due to its detrimental effects on serum lipids, excessive fructose consumption has been discouraged by some health organizations, including the American Diabetes Association, the European Association for the Study of Diabetes, and the AHA.

Chapter 5:
Amazing Recipes

Has your doctor advised you or a loved one to follow a low-purine diet to ease gout's excruciating symptoms? If so, it's critical to comprehend what a low-purine diet is and how it might support your total gout treatment approach in managing your gout. Bringing uric acid levels to a healthy level and maintaining them there is crucial. Without appropriate care, gout flares can increase in frequency, impact additional joints, damage bones, and joints, and result in these and other serious gout consequences.

Breakfast: For some people, this is the meal they look forward to the most each day. As the fast concludes, you can treat yourself to some delectable eggs and bacon, pancakes and waffles, or perhaps a bowl of cereal with honey and chocolate chips on top.

Hmm!

Hold up, though, if you have gout! It's possible that some of the breakfast foods on this list may be unhealthy for you. The majority of them are negative. So nasty that they might quickly raise your uric acid level! I'm not making this up.

The reason of your recent gout attacks can be found by just looking toward what you take for breakfast. Just consider a few of the popular breakfast items of today:

- Eggs

There are several guidelines about eggs that gout sufferers must adhere to. Merely boiled eggs can be eaten because other techniques, including frying, only diminish their excellent health advantages.

It doesn't matter if you cook it in "good" oil like olive oil. Once it's been fried, the amount of free radicals increases, further endangering your health. Save yourself the trouble, then, and limit your egg consumption to simply a few times each week— no more than six—going forward. The good news is that you can eat the entire egg when you prepare it this way, including the yolk! You truly aren't missing out on anything because the egg yolk contains more vitamins and minerals than the egg white. Boiling eggs can be used in salads, sandwiches, dips, and other dishes. Just use your imagination.

- Oatmeal

Oatmeal is a filling breakfast option despite having some purines in it. Whatever your uric acid level, if you pick the correct oatmeal and toppings, you may be protected from gout attacks and able to make use of its excellent benefits.

Minerals like manganese, phosphorus, copper, biotin, chromium, magnesium, and molybdenum are present in oatmeal. It improves immunological response, lowers cholesterol, and stabilizes blood sugar levels. Additionally, oatmeal has laxative properties that support a regular flow of food through your body.

• Having coffee is healthy. The world's favorite beverage is certainly coffee. Some individuals believe they cannot begin their day without their morning caffeine fix. The good news is that you can drink coffee if you fall into this category. It is advised since coffee may help with gout.

In one 12-year study, men over the age of 40 were the subjects. They were interested in learning whether coffee has any impact on reducing gout risk. They discovered that people who drank more coffee had a lower risk of having a gout attack. The lowest risk was actually among people who drank more than six cups of coffee per day!

This is due to chlorogenic acid, an antioxidant found in coffee that may lower uric acid and insulin levels. You can prevent those awful gout attacks as a result.

One restriction is that coffee only reduces risk in people who haven't yet contracted the disease. If you already have gout but you don't often drink coffee, The results may not be as dramatic.

- avoid artificial sugars.

The first thing that springs to mind is orange juice. Okay, if you manufacture your juice. But if it's from a store, it probably contains a lot of sugar, especially high fructose sugar, which is terrible for your health.

Additionally, there are those breakfast options that appear to be healthy, such as smoothies and smoothie bowls, but which, if you're not cautious, can contain a lot of extra sweets, like chocolate chips, dried fruit, almond milk, honey, etc. When you purchase those smoothies from a store, it is worse. There is no way to know what is actually in your food if you are not the one creating it.

- Why are sugars and fructose causing us such concern?

Fructose causes the release of substances known as purines, which may enhance the body's synthesis of uric acid. Therefore, in addition to expanding your girth, you also raise your risk of experiencing a gout attack. No, I mean it. Effects happen very quickly. Once you consume that sugary beverage, your uric acid level quickly increases as well. This extends beyond beverages. Donuts, muffins, and granola bars, which are not at all considered real food, are some people's go-to morning meals. Sorry to burst your bubble, but these are sugar bombs that will cause a terrible crash after giving you a little thrill in the morning.

In essence, you're having cake for breakfast. If you're not a five-year-old, you should not treat your body that way.

Don't ever consume it for breakfast if it isn't fruit juice you made yourself or a smoothie with a higher veggie-to-fruit ratio. You should try to limit your intake of sugar because gout is closely related to diseases that affect your blood sugar, like diabetes and metabolic syndrome. They are connected in that your risk for hyperuricemia rises if your body doesn't react properly to insulin. Additionally, you are more likely to be insulin resistant if you have hyperuricemia.

All of this may seem fruitless, but it is the reality. If you want to, you can occasionally treat yourself to a lovely muffin for breakfast, but only as a treat. Your body will start to crave these sweet foods less as you consume fewer of them. And the more you fill up on actual nutritious meals, the more accustomed your taste buds will become to them; in fact, they may even come to like them because you won't be exposed to the strong, artificial flavors that

manufacturers put in these
unhealthy snacks.

Lunch and dinner:
- One-Pot Chicken and Lentil
  Stew :

Celery reduces inflammation,
lentils are low in purines, which
can trigger gout flare-ups, and
yogurt and lean meats like
chicken are suggested in a gout-
prone diet. These are the main
ingredients in this stew.
- Chicken Broccoli Casserole
  with Cherries and Almonds.

Cherries' anti-inflammatory
properties can help with gout, and

they also give this hearty casserole a sweet, tart touch.

Quinoa Tofu Tacos

Tofu is a preferred source of protein because the majority of the purine content in soy products is removed during the production process. For some clients, moving to plant-based protein choices like tofu can be intimidating. Tacos and chili are two delicious meals to include into. They can add their preferred toppings to this delectable, adaptable meal that is full of fiber and protein.

- Meat swaps

Meat is one of the main dietary factors that raise uric acid levels. Purines are abundant in animal proteins, particularly organ meats like the liver. It's a good idea to eat less meat overall if you have gout. Try to fill out more of your plate with plant-based foods and serve high-protein dishes as a side dish or appetizer. And a lot more.....

Drinks and snacks

- Water:

 Eight glasses of water a day are necessary for gout sufferers as more water is required to minimize swelling brought on by the condition. Water flushes uric acid from the body and moisturizes the joints to avert severe disease and uric acid crystallization.Clear fluids: Broth or herbal teas (bought from reliable sources, such as chamomile, lavender, green, and hibiscus) are alternative options for upping your fluid intake. So, boosting fluid intake is crucial to combating gout symptoms.

Coffee:

Coffee may help the body produce less uric acid. Gout sufferers must also drink coffee with moderate or skimmed milk without sugar to prevent attacks. The recommended amount of coffee is one to two glasses..

• Lemon water:

A study found that drinking lemon water or other liquids high in vitamin C could assist the body in neutralizing uric acid. Squeezing two fresh lemons into 2 liters of drinking water will aid in lowering uric acid levels within the body. Apparently orange juice has medicinal benefits, but only when used in balance..

- Fresh cherry juice:

Fresh cherry juice contains anti-inflammatory antioxidants called anthocyanins that lessen inflammation related to gout. A study found that drinking cherry juice for two days dramatically reduces the signs and symptoms of gout..

- Skimmed milk:

often known as low-fat milk, may help to lower uric acid levels in the body. Thus, consuming low-fat yogurt or skim milk can reduce the incidence of gout attacks.

- Wine:

Generally speaking, drinking can make arthritic symptoms worse. As a result, a doctor may advise you to moderate your alcohol consumption. The least offensive option, if you still want to consume alcohol, seems to be wine. Various types of alcohol have a high purine content, which exacerbates the symptoms of gout.

Green tea:

Studies show that drinking green tea slightly lowers uric acid levels in the blood. Its antioxidant qualities might aid in reducing gout-related inflammation. More evidence is yet required to support these claims. Drinking green tea may have positive overall effects.

Conclusion:

Arthritis and other health problems can be brought on by high levels of uric acid in the body. When our body can't get rid of waste, uric acid levels rise and the body produces gout, which is characterized by solid crystals in the joints. Maintaining one's health is crucial, just like with any other health concern. Eating a balanced diet that contains all the necessary nutrients, such as carbs, proteins, good and healthy fatty acids, vitamins, and minerals, is necessary. Choosing nourishing foods for their diets might be difficult for those with high blood levels of uric acid. However some gout sufferers benefit from treatment, dietary and lifestyle changes could also be helpful. Lowering uric acid can lower the likelihood of developing the illness and may potentially stop flare-ups.

Gout risk, however, is influenced by more than just lifestyle choices. Obesity, being a man and having particular medical conditions are risk factors.

Manufactured by Amazon.ca
Acheson, AB

13436774R00055